Complete Anti-Inflammatory Diet Cookbook Guide

A Complete Stress-Free Meal Plan To Anti-Inflammatory Diet Featuring Simple Recipes To Support Immune Health Alongside A 14-Day Healthy Meal Schedule

Ryan Weimann Bailey

Table of Contents

Introduction

Inflammation stands as a cornerstone of the body's intricate defense mechanisms, an awe-inspiring symphony orchestrated by the immune system in response to threats and challenges faced by our biological system. This intricate process is not just a singular event but a multi-faceted and dynamic defense strategy aimed at safeguarding our well-being.

At its core, inflammation acts as a sentinel, swiftly mobilizing a diverse array of cells, proteins, and chemical messengers in a synchronized effort to address any perceived danger. It's a finely choreographed dance where immune cells such as macrophages, neutrophils, and lymphocytes take center stage, guided by signaling molecules like cytokines and chemokines.

When a threat is detected—be it a cut, an invading pathogen, or an abnormal cell—this immune response is triggered. It's akin to a red alert, prompting the body's blood vessels to dilate and become more permeable, facilitating the arrival of immune cells to the battleground. This influx of cells, along with an increase in blood flow, manifests as the telltale signs of inflammation: warmth, redness, swelling, and sometimes discomfort.

However, this seemingly chaotic commotion is a well-orchestrated defense mechanism. The goal is not just to isolate and neutralize the threat but also to initiate the repair and healing process. Cells work tirelessly to clear away debris and damaged tissue while initiating the regeneration of healthy cells, fostering an environment conducive to recovery.

Moreover, inflammation isn't confined to a localized response; it's a systemic phenomenon with far-reaching implications for the entire body. It communicates with different organs and systems, orchestrating a coordinated effort to ensure the body's overall protection.

In essence, inflammation is the body's vigilant guardian, an evolutionary marvel honed over millennia to shield us from harm. Its intricate dance of cells and molecules is a testament to the remarkable resilience and adaptability of the human body, demonstrating a profound ability to respond and adapt to the ever-changing challenges it encounters.

Benefits of an Anti-Inflammatory Diet

An anti-inflammatory diet offers a myriad of benefits that extend far beyond just reducing inflammation. Here are some key advantages:

Reduction of Chronic Inflammation:

Foremost, an anti-inflammatory diet aims to mitigate chronic inflammation, which is linked to numerous diseases like heart disease, diabetes, arthritis, and certain cancers. By curbing this persistent low-grade inflammation, it helps lower the risk of developing these conditions.

Supports Overall Heart Health: This diet tends to be rich in heart-healthy foods like fruits, vegetables, whole grains, and healthy fats (such as those found in nuts, seeds, and fatty fish). It can help lower cholesterol levels, decrease blood pressure, and reduce the risk of cardiovascular diseases.

Improved Gut Health: Anti-inflammatory foods, particularly those high in fiber and probiotics (like yogurt and fermented foods), support a healthy gut microbiome. A balanced gut microbiota is associated with better digestion, enhanced nutrient absorption, and a stronger immune system.

Weight Management: Emphasizing whole, nutrient-dense foods over processed options can aid in weight management. These foods tend to be more filling, helping to control appetite and reduce overeating, which in turn can contribute to maintaining a healthy weight.

Enhanced Brain Health: Some components of an anti-inflammatory diet, such as omega-3 fatty acids found in fish, nuts, and seeds, are beneficial for brain health. They may reduce the risk of cognitive decline and support better mental health.

Balanced Blood Sugar Levels: Whole, unprocessed foods with a low glycemic index, like vegetables, whole grains, and legumes, can help stabilize blood sugar levels. This is particularly beneficial for individuals with diabetes or those at risk of developing it.

Boosts Immune Function: Certain nutrients present in anti-inflammatory foods, such as vitamins A, C, and E, as well as zinc and selenium, support immune function. A diet rich in these nutrients can help strengthen the immune system and improve the body's ability to fight infections.

Reduced Joint Pain: For individuals with inflammatory conditions like rheumatoid arthritis or osteoarthritis, adopting an anti-inflammatory diet may help alleviate joint pain and stiffness by reducing inflammation in the body.

Promotes Longevity and Overall Well-Being: By reducing the risk of chronic diseases, supporting organ health, and providing a rich array of nutrients, an anti-inflammatory diet contributes to a healthier and more vibrant life, potentially extending longevity.

CHAPTER ONE

The Basics of an Anti-Inflammatory Diet

An anti-inflammatory diet is centered around consuming foods that have the potential to reduce chronic inflammation in the body. It emphasizes whole, nutrient-dense foods while minimizing or avoiding processed and pro-inflammatory options. The focus lies on incorporating a variety of fruits, vegetables, healthy fats, lean proteins, and whole grains.

Foods to Include

Colorful Fruits and Vegetables: Berries, leafy greens, tomatoes, peppers, and other brightly colored fruits and vegetables are rich in antioxidants and phytonutrients, known for their anti-inflammatory properties.

Healthy Fats: Sources like olive oil, avocados, nuts, and seeds provide monounsaturated and polyunsaturated fats, including omega-3 fatty acids. These fats help reduce inflammation and support heart health.

Fatty Fish: Salmon, mackerel, sardines, and other fatty fish are abundant in omega-3s, which have potent anti-inflammatory effects.

Whole Grains: Quinoa, brown rice, barley, and whole wheat are examples of whole grains that offer fiber and nutrients, contributing to a balanced diet and potentially reducing inflammation.

Legumes: Beans, lentils, and chickpeas are excellent sources of plant-based protein, fiber, and antioxidants, offering anti-inflammatory benefits.

Herbs and Spices: Turmeric, ginger, garlic, cinnamon, and other spices contain compounds with anti-inflammatory properties and can be used to flavor dishes.

Foods to Avoid

Processed Foods: Highly processed foods often contain unhealthy fats, added sugars, and artificial additives that can promote inflammation. This includes fast food, sugary snacks, and processed meats.

Trans Fats and Saturated Fats: Foods high in trans fats and saturated fats, like fried foods, margarine, and fatty cuts of meat, can contribute to inflammation.

Refined Carbohydrates: White bread, pastries, and sugary cereals are examples of refined carbohydrates that can cause spikes in blood sugar levels and promote inflammation.

Excessive Sugar: Added sugars, often found in soda, candy, and many processed foods, can lead to increased inflammation when consumed in excess.

Highly Processed Oils: Vegetable oils high in omega-6 fatty acids, such as soybean oil and corn oil, when consumed in large quantities, can contribute to inflammation.

Building Blocks of Anti-Inflammatory Cooking

Healthy Cooking Methods: Emphasize cooking techniques like steaming, sautéing in healthy oils, roasting, and grilling to retain the nutrients in foods without adding excess unhealthy fats.

Experiment with Herbs and Spices: Incorporate flavorful herbs and spices known for their anti-inflammatory properties into your meals to enhance taste while promoting health.

Focus on Whole Foods: Strive to include a variety of whole, unprocessed foods in your meals to maximize nutrient intake and minimize exposure to pro-inflammatory additives.

Mindful Eating: Pay attention to portion sizes and listen to your body's hunger and fullness cues to maintain a balanced and nourishing diet.

CHAPTER TWO

Breakfast

Energizing Morning Smoothies

Start your day with vibrant, nutrient-packed smoothies that provide a burst of energy while supporting an anti-inflammatory diet. Here are a few recipes to consider:

Green Goddess Smoothie

Ingredients: Spinach, kale, banana, pineapple, ginger, coconut water.

Benefits: Packed with antioxidants, vitamins, and anti-inflammatory compounds from leafy greens and ginger.

Berry Blast Smoothie

Ingredients: Mixed berries (blueberries, strawberries, raspberries), almond milk, chia seeds, spinach.

Benefits: Rich in antioxidants, fiber, and omega-3 fatty acids from chia seeds.

Tropical Turmeric Smoothie

Ingredients: Mango, pineapple, turmeric, Greek yogurt, coconut milk.

Benefits: Turmeric's anti-inflammatory properties combined with tropical fruits for a refreshing start.

Anti-Inflammatory Breakfast Bowls

These breakfast bowls offer a hearty and nourishing way to kickstart your morning with anti-inflammatory ingredients:

Quinoa Breakfast Bowl

Ingredients: Cooked quinoa, mixed berries, walnuts, honey or maple syrup, cinnamon.

Benefits: Quinoa provides protein and fiber while berries and nuts offer antioxidants and healthy fats.

Chia Seed Pudding Bowl

Ingredients: Chia seeds, almond milk, sliced almonds, diced mango or kiwi, shredded coconut.

Benefits: Chia seeds are rich in omega-3s and fiber, complemented by the fruit's vitamins and minerals.

Sweet Potato Breakfast Bowl

Ingredients: Roasted sweet potato cubes, Greek yogurt, granola, drizzle of honey, cinnamon.

Benefits: Sweet potatoes provide antioxidants and fiber, paired with the probiotics in Greek yogurt.

Creative Grain-Free Pancakes and Waffles

Enjoy breakfast favorites without grains, focusing on nutrient-dense alternatives:

Almond Flour Pancakes

Ingredients: Almond flour, eggs, almond milk, vanilla extract.

Benefits: Almond flour offers protein and healthy fats while being grain-free and low in carbohydrates.

Coconut Flour Waffles

Ingredients: Coconut flour, eggs, coconut milk, baking powder.

Benefits: Coconut flour is high in fiber and supports a gluten-free, anti-inflammatory approach.

Banana-Oat Pancakes (Optional Grain Inclusion)

Ingredients: Mashed banana, oats, eggs, cinnamon.

Benefits: Offers a slight grain inclusion while bananas provide potassium and fiber.

CHAPTER THREE

Lunches

Wholesome Salads and Dressings

Create vibrant salads packed with nutrients and pair them with homemade dressings that accentuate flavor while adhering to an anti-inflammatory diet:

Kale and Quinoa Salad

Ingredients: Massaged kale, cooked quinoa, cherry tomatoes, cucumber, avocado, toasted pumpkin seeds.

Dressing: Lemon-tahini dressing (tahini, lemon juice, garlic, olive oil).

Benefits: High in antioxidants, fiber, and healthy fats from kale, quinoa, and avocado.

Mediterranean Chickpea Salad

Ingredients: Chickpeas, chopped cucumber, bell peppers, red onion, olives, feta cheese (optional).

Dressing: Olive oil, balsamic vinegar, garlic, oregano, lemon juice.

Benefits: Protein and fiber-rich from chickpeas, paired with flavorful Mediterranean ingredients.

Asian-Inspired Rainbow Salad

Ingredients: Shredded cabbage, carrots, bell peppers, edamame, mandarin oranges.

Dressing: Ginger-sesame dressing (ginger, sesame oil, rice vinegar, soy sauce).

Benefits: Colorful mix packed with vitamins, minerals, and plant-based protein from edamame.

Hearty Soups and Stews

Warm, comforting bowls of soup and stew can be nutrient-dense while incorporating anti-inflammatory ingredients:

Turmeric Lentil Soup

Ingredients: Red lentils, carrots, celery, onions, turmeric, cumin.

Benefits: Turmeric's anti-inflammatory properties combined with fiber and protein from lentils.

Vegetable Quinoa Soup

Ingredients: Mixed vegetables (zucchini, spinach, tomatoes), quinoa, vegetable broth.

Benefits: Quinoa adds protein, while vegetables offer an array of vitamins and antioxidants.

Chicken and Vegetable Stew

Ingredients: Chicken breast, sweet potatoes, bell peppers, kale, garlic, chicken broth.

Benefits: Protein-rich chicken combined with colorful vegetables for a hearty, wholesome stew.

Flavorful Wraps and Sandwiches

Create satisfying wraps and sandwiches using wholesome ingredients and inventive combinations:

Mediterranean Veggie Wrap

Ingredients: Hummus, roasted vegetables (eggplant, bell peppers, zucchini), feta cheese, spinach, whole-grain wrap.

Benefits: Loads of fiber, vitamins, and healthy fats from vegetables and hummus.

Grilled Chicken and Avocado Sandwich

Ingredients: Grilled chicken breast, avocado slices, mixed greens, whole-grain bread.

Benefits: Lean protein from chicken and healthy fats from avocado in a filling sandwich.

Salmon Salad Lettuce Wraps

Ingredients: Flaked salmon, Greek yogurt, dill, cucumber, lettuce leaves.

Benefits: Omega-3s from salmon paired with refreshing cucumber and yogurt dressing.

CHAPTER FOUR

Satisfying Dinners

Vibrant Vegetable Stir-Fries

Stir-fries are a fantastic way to incorporate an array of colorful veggies while keeping the flavors vibrant and the nutrients intact:

Rainbow Vegetable Stir-Fry

Ingredients: Bell peppers, broccoli, snow peas, carrots, mushrooms, tofu or tempeh.

Sauce: Ginger-garlic sauce (ginger, garlic, soy sauce, sesame oil).

Benefits: High in fiber, antioxidants, and plant-based protein from vegetables and tofu/tempeh.

Spicy Chickpea Stir-Fry

Ingredients: Chickpeas, spinach, bell peppers, onions, cauliflower, curry spices.

Sauce: Tomato-based sauce with turmeric, cumin, and paprika.

Benefits: Protein and fiber-rich chickpeas with a flavorful, anti-inflammatory spice blend.

Sesame Ginger Tofu Stir-Fry

Ingredients: Tofu, bok choy, snap peas, bell peppers, broccoli.

Sauce: Sesame-ginger sauce (sesame oil, ginger, garlic, soy sauce).

Benefits: Tofu provides protein while vegetables offer an array of vitamins and minerals.

Protein-Packed Main Dishes

Incorporate lean protein sources and anti-inflammatory ingredients into satisfying main courses:

Baked Salmon with Herbed Quinoa

Ingredients: Baked salmon fillets, quinoa cooked with fresh herbs (parsley, dill), lemon zest.

Benefits: Omega-3s from salmon combined with protein and nutrients from quinoa and herbs.

Turkey and Vegetable Skewers

Ingredients: Turkey breast cubes, bell peppers, red onions, cherry tomatoes.

Marinade: Olive oil, garlic, lemon juice, oregano.

Benefits: Lean protein from turkey with a burst of flavor from the marinade and veggies.

Eggplant and Lentil Moussaka

Ingredients: Layers of eggplant, lentil-based filling, tomato sauce, topped with yogurt.

Benefits: Fiber and protein from lentils, along with vitamins and antioxidants from eggplant and tomatoes.

Comforting One-Pot Meals

These cozy and wholesome one-pot meals offer convenience and a fusion of flavors:

Vegetable and Chickpea Curry

Ingredients: Chickpeas, mixed vegetables, coconut milk, curry spices.

Benefits: Protein-rich chickpeas with a medley of vegetables in a creamy, flavorful sauce.

Quinoa and Black Bean Chili

Ingredients: Quinoa, black beans, tomatoes, bell peppers, chili spices.

Benefits: Protein and fiber from black beans and quinoa, with a punch of antioxidants from vegetables.

Chicken and Vegetable Brown Rice Pilaf

Ingredients: Chicken thighs, brown rice, mixed veggies, chicken broth, herbs.

Benefits: Whole grains in brown rice, lean protein from chicken, and a mix of vitamins from vegetables.

CHAPTER FIVE

Side Dishes and Snacks

Colorful Veggie Sides

Enhance your meals with vibrant and nutritious vegetable sides that add a pop of color and nutrients:

Roasted Garlic Brussels Sprouts

Ingredients: Brussels sprouts, garlic cloves, olive oil, balsamic vinegar.

Benefits: Brussels sprouts offer antioxidants and fiber while garlic adds flavor and potential anti-inflammatory properties.

Turmeric-Roasted Carrots

Ingredients: Carrots, turmeric, honey, olive oil, cumin.

Benefits: Carrots are rich in beta-carotene, paired with turmeric's anti-inflammatory properties.

Sautéed Spinach with Garlic and Lemon

Ingredients: Fresh spinach, garlic, lemon juice, olive oil.

Benefits: Spinach is packed with vitamins and iron, complemented by the tangy zest of lemon.

Nutritious Snack Ideas

Snack time can be both delicious and nutritious by incorporating whole foods and flavorsome combinations:

Almond Butter and Apple Slices

Benefits: Apples provide fiber and antioxidants while almond butter offers healthy fats and protein.

Greek Yogurt Parfait with Berries

Ingredients: Greek yogurt, mixed berries, a drizzle of honey or a sprinkle of nuts/seeds.

Benefits: Protein-rich yogurt combined with antioxidants and fiber from fresh berries.

Homemade Trail Mix

Ingredients: Mixed nuts, seeds (like pumpkin or sunflower), dried fruits (cranberries, apricots), dark chocolate chips.

Benefits: Nuts and seeds offer healthy fats and protein, while dried fruits add natural sweetness.

Homemade Dips and Spreads

Elevate your meals with flavorful homemade dips and spreads that are versatile and full of healthful ingredients:

Avocado Hummus

Ingredients: Chickpeas, avocado, tahini, garlic, lemon juice.

Benefits: Creamy avocado provides healthy fats and nutrients alongside protein-rich chickpeas.

Roasted Red Pepper Dip

Ingredients: Roasted red peppers, Greek yogurt, garlic, paprika, olive oil.

Benefits: Red peppers offer antioxidants, while Greek yogurt adds probiotics and protein.

Herbed Cottage Cheese Spread

Ingredients: Cottage cheese, fresh herbs (parsley, chives), lemon zest, black pepper.

Benefits: Cottage cheese provides protein and calcium, while fresh herbs add flavor and nutrients.

CHAPTER SIX

Sweet Treats

Guilt-Free Desserts

Indulge in desserts that satisfy your sweet tooth without compromising on health:

Chia Seed Pudding

Ingredients: Chia seeds, coconut milk, vanilla extract, fresh fruit toppings.

Benefits: Chia seeds offer omega-3s and fiber, paired with the natural sweetness of fruits.

Dark Chocolate Covered Berries

Ingredients: Fresh berries (strawberries, blueberries) dipped in melted dark chocolate.

Benefits: Dark chocolate contains antioxidants and can satisfy chocolate cravings in moderation.

Baked Apples with Cinnamon

Ingredients: Sliced apples sprinkled with cinnamon, baked until tender.

Benefits: Apples provide fiber and antioxidants, while cinnamon adds flavor without extra sugar.

Healthy Baking and Dessert Swaps

Revamp traditional dessert recipes with healthier ingredient alternatives:

Oat Flour Banana Bread

Ingredients: Oat flour, ripe bananas, Greek yogurt, a touch of honey or maple syrup.

Benefits: Oat flour adds fiber, and ripe bananas offer natural sweetness.

Coconut Flour Blueberry Muffins

Ingredients: Coconut flour, eggs, almond milk, fresh blueberries.

Benefits: Coconut flour is gluten-free and adds fiber, while blueberries offer antioxidants.

Almond Flour Chocolate Chip Cookies

Ingredients: Almond flour, dark chocolate chips, coconut oil, a touch of coconut sugar.

Benefits: Almond flour provides protein and healthy fats, while dark chocolate adds antioxidants.

Decadent Fruit-Based Sweets

Enjoy the natural sweetness of fruits in delightful dessert options:

Grilled Pineapple with Cinnamon

Ingredients: Pineapple slices grilled and dusted with cinnamon.

Benefits: Pineapple contains bromelain, an enzyme with potential anti-inflammatory properties.

Frozen Banana "Nice Cream"

Ingredients: Frozen bananas blended until creamy, topped with nuts or dark chocolate.

Benefits: Bananas provide potassium and natural sweetness without added sugar.

Mixed Berry Sorbet

Ingredients: Blend of frozen mixed berries with a splash of lemon juice.

Benefits: Berries are rich in antioxidants and vitamins, offering a refreshing dessert option.

CHAPTER SEVEN

Beverages and Drinks

Rejuvenating Teas and Infusions

These comforting and beneficial teas and infusions can be a part of a relaxing routine:

Turmeric-Ginger Tea

Ingredients: Fresh turmeric, ginger slices, boiling water.

Benefits: Both turmeric and ginger possess anti-inflammatory properties, making this a soothing and health-boosting infusion.

Chamomile-Lavender Tea

Ingredients: Dried chamomile flowers, lavender buds, hot water.

Benefits: Chamomile and lavender are known for their calming effects and can aid in reducing stress, potentially lowering inflammation.

Green Tea with Citrus

Ingredients: Green tea leaves, lemon or orange slices.

Benefits: Green tea is rich in antioxidants and pairing it with citrus adds a refreshing twist while enhancing the benefits.

Hydrating Smoothies and Juices

Nourish your body with hydrating and nutrient-packed beverages:

Cucumber-Mint Hydrating Juice

Ingredients: Cucumber, mint leaves, a splash of lime juice.

Benefits: Cucumbers are hydrating, and mint offers a refreshing taste with potential digestive benefits.

Berry-Beet Antioxidant Smoothie

Ingredients: Mixed berries, cooked beets, coconut water.

Benefits: Berries are rich in antioxidants, while beets offer vitamins and potential anti-inflammatory compounds.

Pineapple-Turmeric Immune Booster

Ingredients: Pineapple chunks, turmeric root, coconut water or almond milk.

Benefits: Pineapple contains bromelain, and turmeric offers anti-inflammatory properties, boosting overall immunity.

Herbal Tonics and Elixirs

These concoctions can be both invigorating and health-enhancing:

Elderberry-Echinacea Tonic

Ingredients: Elderberries, echinacea, honey, boiling water.

Benefits: Both elderberry and echinacea are believed to support the immune system.

Ashwagandha-Adaptogen Elixir

Ingredients: Ashwagandha powder, adaptogenic herbs, almond milk, honey.

Benefits: Ashwagandha is an adaptogenic herb known for its potential stress-reducing effects.

Nettle-Lemon Detox Elixir

Ingredients: Nettle tea infusion, lemon juice, a touch of honey.

Benefits: Nettle is believed to support detoxification and may have anti-inflammatory properties.

CHAPTER EIGHT

Weekly Meal Plans and Recipes

Sample Meal Plan:

Day 1:

Breakfast:

Berry Blast Smoothie: Mixed berries, chia seeds, spinach, almond milk.

Lunch:

Mediterranean Chickpea Salad: Chickpeas, cucumbers, bell peppers, feta cheese, olives, olive oil-lemon dressing.

Snack:

Almond Butter and Apple Slices: Sliced apple with almond butter.

Dinner:

Turmeric Lentil Soup: Red lentils, carrots, onions, turmeric, cumin.

Day 2:

Breakfast:

Avocado Toast: Whole-grain toast topped with mashed avocado, tomato slices, and a sprinkle of hemp seeds.

Lunch:

Grilled Chicken and Avocado Sandwich: Grilled chicken breast, avocado, mixed greens on whole-grain bread.

Snack:

Greek Yogurt Parfait with Berries: Greek yogurt, mixed berries, a drizzle of honey.

Dinner:

Rainbow Vegetable Stir-Fry: Mixed vegetables, tofu, ginger-garlic sauce, served with quinoa.

Recipes for Each Meal:

Breakfast:

Green Goddess Smoothie: Spinach, kale, banana, pineapple, coconut water.

Oat Flour Banana Bread: Oat flour, ripe bananas, Greek yogurt, a touch of honey.

Lunch:

Quinoa Lunch Bowl: Quinoa, mixed veggies, chickpeas, lemon-tahini dressing.

Coconut Flour Blueberry Muffins: Coconut flour, eggs, almond milk, fresh blueberries.

Dinner:

Baked Salmon with Herbed Quinoa: Salmon fillets, quinoa cooked with herbs, lemon zest.

Vegetable and Chickpea Curry: Chickpeas, mixed veggies, coconut milk, curry spices.

Snacks:

Dark Chocolate Covered Berries: Fresh berries dipped in melted dark chocolate.

Chia Seed Pudding: Chia seeds, coconut milk, vanilla extract, topped with fresh fruits.

14 days Sample Meal Plans

Here are two weeks' worth of sample meal plans focusing on an anti-inflammatory approach:

Day 1:

Breakfast:

Berry Blast Smoothie: Mixed berries, chia seeds, spinach, almond milk.

Lunch:

Mediterranean Chickpea Salad: Chickpeas, cucumbers, bell peppers, feta cheese, olives, olive oil-lemon dressing.

Snack:

Almond Butter and Apple Slices: Sliced apple with almond butter.

Dinner:

Turmeric Lentil Soup: Red lentils, carrots, onions, turmeric, cumin.

Day 2:

Breakfast:

Avocado Toast: Whole-grain toast topped with mashed avocado, tomato slices, and a sprinkle of hemp seeds.

Lunch:

Grilled Chicken and Avocado Sandwich: Grilled chicken breast, avocado, mixed greens on whole-grain bread.

Snack:

Greek Yogurt Parfait with Berries: Greek yogurt, mixed berries, a drizzle of honey.

Dinner:

Rainbow Vegetable Stir-Fry: Mixed vegetables, tofu, ginger-garlic sauce, served with quinoa.

Day 3:

Breakfast:

Green Goddess Smoothie: Spinach, kale, banana, pineapple, coconut water.

Lunch:

Quinoa Lunch Bowl: Quinoa, mixed veggies, chickpeas, lemon-tahini dressing.

Snack:

Dark Chocolate Covered Berries: Fresh berries dipped in melted dark chocolate.

Dinner:

Baked Salmon with Herbed Quinoa: Salmon fillets, quinoa cooked with herbs, lemon zest.

Day 4:

Breakfast:

Oat Flour Banana Bread: Oat flour, ripe bananas, Greek yogurt, a touch of honey.

Lunch:

Coconut Flour Blueberry Muffins: Coconut flour, eggs, almond milk, fresh blueberries.

Snack:

Chia Seed Pudding: Chia seeds, coconut milk, vanilla extract, topped with fresh fruits.

Dinner:

Vegetable and Chickpea Curry: Chickpeas, mixed veggies, coconut milk, curry spices.

Day 5:

Breakfast:

Pineapple-Turmeric Immune Booster: Pineapple chunks, turmeric root, coconut water or almond milk.

Lunch:

Roasted Garlic Brussels Sprouts: Brussels sprouts, garlic cloves, olive oil, balsamic vinegar.

Snack:

Cucumber-Mint Hydrating Juice: Cucumber, mint leaves, a splash of lime juice.

Dinner:

Chicken and Vegetable Brown Rice Pilaf: Chicken thighs, brown rice, mixed veggies, herbs.

Day 6:

Breakfast:

Acai Bowl: Acai puree, banana, mixed berries, topped with granola and shredded coconut.

Lunch:

Spinach and Feta Stuffed Bell Peppers: Bell peppers stuffed with spinach, feta, quinoa, baked.

Snack:

Mixed Nuts and Dried Fruit: A handful of mixed nuts and dried fruits.

Dinner:

Spicy Chickpea Stir-Fry: Chickpeas, spinach, bell peppers, cauliflower, curry spices.

Day 7:

Breakfast:

Green Tea with Citrus: Green tea leaves with lemon or orange slices.

Lunch:

Sweet Potato and Lentil Salad: Roasted sweet potato cubes, lentils, mixed greens, balsamic vinaigrette.

Snack:

Frozen Banana "Nice Cream": Frozen bananas blended until creamy, topped with nuts or dark chocolate.

Dinner:

Mediterranean Baked Cod: Cod fillets baked with tomatoes, olives, and herbs, served with quinoa.

Day 8:

Breakfast:

Chia Seed Pudding: Chia seeds, almond milk, topped with fresh fruits and a drizzle of honey.

Lunch:

Tuna Salad Lettuce Wraps: Tuna salad with Greek yogurt, celery, wrapped in lettuce leaves.

Snack:

Homemade Trail Mix: Mixed nuts, seeds, and a few dark chocolate chips.

Dinner:

Eggplant and Lentil Moussaka: Layers of eggplant, lentil filling, tomato sauce, baked until golden.

Day 9:

Breakfast:

Coconut Flour Pancakes: Coconut flour, eggs, almond milk, topped with fresh berries.

Lunch:

Quinoa and Black Bean Chili: Quinoa, black beans, tomatoes, bell peppers, chili spices.

Snack:

Mixed Berry Sorbet: Blend of frozen mixed berries with a splash of lemon juice.

Dinner:

Grilled Turkey Skewers with Veggie Medley: Turkey breast cubes, mixed veggies, grilled and served with a side salad.

Day 10:

Breakfast:

Greek Yogurt Parfait with Berries: Greek yogurt, mixed berries, a sprinkle of granola.

Lunch:

Asian-Inspired Rainbow Salad: Shredded cabbage, carrots, edamame, mandarin oranges, sesame-ginger dressing.

Snack:

Homemade Hummus with Veggie Sticks: Carrot and cucumber sticks with hummus.

Dinner:

Salmon Salad Lettuce Wraps: Flaked salmon, Greek yogurt, dill, cucumber, wrapped in lettuce leaves.

Day 11:

Breakfast:

Almond Flour Chocolate Chip Cookies: Almond flour, dark chocolate chips, coconut oil.

Lunch:

Nettle-Lemon Detox Elixir: Nettle tea infusion with lemon juice.

Snack:

Roasted Red Pepper Dip with Veggie Sticks: Red pepper dip with carrot and bell pepper sticks.

Dinner:

Chickpea and Spinach Coconut Curry: Chickpeas, spinach, coconut milk, curry spices, served with brown rice.

Day 12:

Breakfast:

Frozen Berry Smoothie Bowl: Frozen berries, banana, almond milk, topped with granola and shredded coconut.

Lunch:

Turkey and Veggie Lettuce Wraps: Sliced turkey, mixed veggies, wrapped in lettuce leaves.

Snack:

Herbed Cottage Cheese Spread with Whole-Grain Crackers: Cottage cheese mixed with fresh herbs, served with crackers.

Dinner:

Stuffed Bell Peppers with Quinoa and Veggies: Bell peppers stuffed with quinoa, veggies, baked until tender.

Day 13:

Breakfast:

Pineapple-Turmeric Immune Booster: Pineapple chunks, turmeric root, coconut water or almond milk.

Lunch:

Chicken and Vegetable Brown Rice Bowl: Grilled chicken, mixed veggies, brown rice, drizzled with soy-ginger sauce.

Snack:

Mixed Nuts Trail Mix: Assorted nuts and seeds with a touch of dried fruit.

Dinner:

Miso-Glazed Eggplant with Tofu:
Roasted eggplant slices, marinated tofu,
served with quinoa.

Day 14:

Breakfast:

Acai Bowl: Acai puree, banana, mixed
berries, topped with granola and
shredded coconut.

Lunch:

Greek Salad with Grilled Chicken: Mixed
greens, tomatoes, cucumber, olives,
feta cheese, grilled chicken, olive oil-
lemon dressing.

Snack:

Homemade Trail Mix: Mixed nuts, seeds, and a few dark chocolate chips.

Dinner:

Baked Cod with Lemon-Herb Quinoa: Cod fillets baked with lemon and herbs, served alongside herbed quinoa.

Conclusion

Adopting an anti-inflammatory diet involves incorporating a diverse range of nutrient-dense foods while minimizing processed and inflammatory-inducing ingredients. This style of eating focuses on whole, natural foods that are rich in antioxidants, healthy fats, fiber, and phytonutrients.

Throughout this sample meal plan, a variety of recipes for breakfast, lunch, dinner, snacks, and beverages have been provided. These recipes emphasize ingredients known for their potential anti-inflammatory properties, such as turmeric, ginger, leafy greens, berries, nuts, seeds, and omega-3-rich foods like salmon.

The goal of this meal plan is to not only promote a healthier lifestyle but also provide delicious and satisfying meal options. By incorporating these recipes and meal ideas into your routine, you can create a balanced and flavorful diet that supports overall well-being and may potentially reduce inflammation.

Remember, individual nutritional needs vary, so it's essential to tailor meal plans to suit personal preferences, dietary restrictions, and health goals. Consulting with a healthcare professional or a registered dietitian can offer personalized guidance for an anti-inflammatory diet suited to your specific needs and health status.

THE END

www.ingramcontent.com/pod-product-compliance
Lightning Source LLC
Chambersburg PA
CBHW050652250726
48662CB00002B/637